A Real Mom's Story: Parenting Manual for ADHD Children, Become the Greatest Parents and Create a Successful Home

Vick West

Table of Contents

CHAPTER 1

A REAL MOM'S STORY

"At the point when Jane initially figured out that her child, Billy, had ADHD, she was overpowered and uncertain of what to do. She had perused all the nurturing books and heeded all the guidance, however nothing appeared to work. She felt like a disappointment, and she didn't have the foggiest idea how to help her child. However, she wouldn't surrender. She realize that there must be a method for aiding her child and to be a fruitful parent. What's more, with a ton of experimentation, she at long last figured out how to help.

Something that Jane acknowledged was that she expected to zero in on building areas of strength for a with her child. She chipped away at building trust, understanding, and correspondence. She likewise figured out how to be patient and adaptable, and to celebrate little victories. She quit attempting to change her child, and on second thought zeroed in on assisting him with fostering the abilities and systems he should have been effective. She likewise figured out how to acknowledge that ADHD was a piece of who her child was, and she embraced his one of a kind qualities and gifts.

Jane's way to deal with nurturing was a distinct advantage for her child. With her help, he had the option to flourish. He figured out how to deal with his ADHD side effects, and he started to succeed in school and in different parts of his life. Jane was pleased with her child's advancement, however more significantly, she was glad for the relationship they had constructed. She felt like an effective parent since she had assisted her child with turning into a fruitful individual. Furthermore, she realize that their process was nowhere near finished. She was eager to see what was in store held for them both.

Throughout the long term, Jane and Billy proceeded to learn and become together. Billy confronted difficulties and mishaps, however with his mother's help, he had the option to defeat them. Furthermore, Jane figured out how to acknowledge that nurturing was not a one-size-fits-all undertaking. She proceeded to learn and develop as a parent, and she tracked down better approaches to interface with and support her child. She realize that the excursion could never be finished, however she additionally realize that the prizes merited the work. Above all, she realize that her child was cheerful, solid, and flourishing.

Billy grew up to be a fruitful and balanced grown-up. He had a fruitful profession, and he found an accomplice who cherished and acknowledged him for what his identity was. What's more, in particular, he had major areas of strength for a caring relationship with his mother. They kept on being close, and Jane was thankful for the years they had spent together on their excursion. She realize that it had not forever been simple, however it had been worth the effort. She had tracked down joy and satisfaction as a parent, and she was thankful for the chance to assist her child with turning into the individual he was intended to be.

Jane always remembered the examples she learned on her nurturing venture. She imparted her encounters to different guardians, expecting to help them on their own excursions. She realized that nurturing was difficult, yet she likewise realize that making progress and fulfillment was conceivable. She accepted that all guardians could track down their own interesting way to progress, and she would have liked to help other people track down the way. She likewise realize that her excursion as a parent was rarely genuinely finished. Indeed, even as her child grew up and turned into a grown-up, she would constantly be there to cherish and uphold him.

The tale of Jane and Billy is a demonstration of the force of adoration, tolerance, and constancy. That's what it shows, with the right help, anybody can make progress and satisfaction as a parent. Jane and Billy's process isn't novel, yet it is a strong sign of the strength of the parent-youngster bond. It is an update that the excursion of life as a parent is rarely finished, and that the prizes are dependably worth the work. It is an account of adoration, development, and win, and it fills in as a motivation to guardians all over the place.

CHAPTER 2

THE TRUTH ABOUT KIDS WITH ADHD

ADHD in Children
Do you think your child might have ADHD? Here's how to recognize the signs and symptoms of attention deficit hyperactivity disorder in girls and boys—and get the help you need.

What is ADHD or ADD?
It's normal for children to occasionally forget their homework, daydream during class, act without thinking, or get fidgety at the dinner table. However inattention, impulsivity, and hyperactivity are also signs of attention deficit hyperactivity disorder (ADHD), sometimes known as attention deficit disorder or ADD.

ADHD is a common neurodevelopmental disorder that typically appears in early childhood, usually before the age of seven.

ADHD makes it difficult for children to inhibit their spontaneous responses—responses that can involve everything from movement to speech to attentiveness. We all know kids who can't sit still, who never seem to listen, who don't follow instructions no matter how clearly you present them, or who blurt out inappropriate comments at inappropriate times. Sometimes these children are labeled as troublemakers, or criticized for being lazy and undisciplined. However, they may have ADHD.

Is it normal kid behavior or is it ADHD?
It can be difficult to distinguish between ADHD and normal "kid behavior." If you spot just a few signs, or the symptoms appear only in some situations, it's probably not ADHD. On the other hand, if your child shows a number of ADHD signs and symptoms that are present across all situations—at home, at school, and at play—it's time to take a closer look.

Life with a child with ADHD can be frustrating and overwhelming, but as a parent there is a lot you can do to help control symptoms, overcome daily challenges, and bring greater calm to your family.

Myths and Facts about ADHD
Myth: All kids with ADHD are hyperactive.
Fact: Some children with ADHD are hyperactive, but many others with attention problems are not. Children with ADHD who are inattentive, but not overly active, may appear to be spacey and unmotivated.

Myth: Kids with ADHD can never pay attention.
Fact: Children with ADHD are often able to concentrate on activities they enjoy. But no matter how hard they try, they have trouble maintaining focus when the task at hand is boring or repetitive.

Myth: Kids with ADHD could behave better if they wanted to.

Fact: Children with ADHD may do their best to be good, but still be unable to sit still, stay quiet, or pay attention. They may appear disobedient, but that doesn't mean they're acting out on purpose.

Myth: Kids will eventually grow out of ADHD.

Fact: ADHD often continues into adulthood, so don't wait for your child to outgrow the problem. Treatment can help your child learn to manage and minimize the symptoms.

Myth: Medication is the best treatment option for ADHD.

Fact: Medication is often prescribed for attention deficit disorder, but it might not be the best option for your child. Effective treatment for ADHD also includes education, behavior therapy, support at home and school, exercise, and proper nutrition.

ADHD symptoms
When many people think of attention deficit disorder, they picture an out-of-control kid in constant motion, bouncing off the walls and disrupting everyone around. But the reality is much more complex. Some children with ADHD are hyperactive, while others sit quietly—with their attention miles away. Some put too much focus on a task and have trouble shifting it to something else. Others are only mildly inattentive, but overly impulsive.

The signs and symptoms a child with attention deficit disorder has depend on which characteristics predominate.

Children with ADHD may be:

Inattentive, but not hyperactive or impulsive.

Hyperactive and impulsive, but able to pay attention.
Inattentive, hyperactive, and impulsive (the most common form of ADHD).
Children who only have inattentive symptoms of ADHD are often overlooked, since they're not disruptive. However, the symptoms of inattention have consequences: getting in hot water with parents and teachers for not following directions; underperforming in school; or clashing with other kids over not playing by the rules.

Which one of these children may have ADHD?
A. The hyperactive boy who talks nonstop and can't sit still.
B. The quiet dreamer who sits at her desk and stares off into space.
C. Both.

The correct answer is "C."

ADHD symptoms at different ages
Because we expect very young children to be easily distractible and hyperactive, it's the impulsive behaviors—the dangerous climb, the blurted insult—that often stand out in preschoolers with ADHD. By age four or five, though, most children have learned how to pay attention to others, to sit quietly when instructed to, and not to say everything that pops into their heads. So by the time children reach school age, those with ADHD stand out in all three behaviors: inattentiveness, hyperactivity, and impulsivity.

ADHD in girls
Girls are less likely to be diagnosed and treated for ADHD than boys. Some people even mistakenly believe that the condition only occurs in boys. In actuality, the symptoms of ADHD can look different in girls in ways that make the disorder harder to notice.

Girls with ADHD may not seem as hyperactive, impulsive, or disruptive in class as boys. However, they may quietly struggle with anxiety, forgetfulness, disorganization, and lack of focus. Girls with ADHD may also use better coping strategies to compensate for their difficulties, such as putting in extra effort into their schoolwork.

Many girls don't receive a formal ADHD diagnosis until later in life. By that time, they've likely had to endure the consequences of living with an unrecognized and untreated disorder. These consequences could include problems in school and relationships, as well as low self-confidence or even depression. Getting an early and accurate diagnosis is the best way to ensure your child gets the support she needs

Inattentiveness signs and symptoms of ADHD
It isn't that children with ADHD can't pay attention: when they're doing things they

enjoy or hearing about topics in which they're interested, they have no trouble focusing and staying on task. But when the task is repetitive or boring, they quickly tune out.

Staying on track is another common problem. Children with ADHD often bounce from task to task without completing any of them, or skip necessary steps in procedures. Organizing their schoolwork and their time is harder for them than it is for most children. Kids with ADHD also have trouble concentrating if there are things going on around them; they usually need a calm, quiet environment in order to stay focused.

Symptoms of inattention in children
Your child may:

Have trouble staying focused; be easily distracted or get bored with a task before it's completed.
Appear not to listen when spoken to.

Have difficulty remembering things and following instructions; not pay attention to details or makes careless mistakes.

Have trouble staying organized, planning ahead, and finishing projects.

Frequently lose or misplace homework, books, toys, or other items.

Speak to a Licensed Therapist

BetterHelp is an online therapy service that matches you to licensed, accredited therapists who can help with depression, anxiety, relationships, and more. Take the assessment and get matched with a therapist in as little as 48 hours.

Take Assessment

HelpGuide is user supported. We may earn a commission if you sign up for BetterHelp's services after clicking through from this site.

Learn more

Hyperactivity signs and symptoms of ADHD

The most obvious sign of ADHD is hyperactivity. While many children are naturally quite active, kids with hyperactive symptoms of attention deficit disorder are always moving. They may try to do several things at once, bouncing around from one activity to the next. Even when forced to sit still, which can be very difficult for them, their foot is tapping, their leg is shaking, or their fingers are drumming.

Symptoms of hyperactivity in children
Your child may:

Constantly fidget and squirm.
Have difficulty sitting still, playing quietly, or relaxing.
Move around constantly, often running or climbing inappropriately.
Talk excessively.
Have a quick temper or "short fuse."
Impulsive signs and symptoms of ADHD
The impulsivity of children with ADHD can cause problems with self-control. Because they censor themselves less than other kids do, they'll interrupt conversations, invade other people's space, ask irrelevant

questions in class, make tactless observations, and ask overly personal questions. Instructions like, "Be patient" and "Just wait a little while" are twice as hard for children with ADHD to follow as they are for other youngsters.

Children with impulsive signs and symptoms of ADHD also tend to be moody and to overreact emotionally. As a result, others may start to view the child as disrespectful, weird, or needy.

Symptoms of impulsivity in children
Your child may:

Act without thinking.
Guess, rather than taking time to solve a problem; blurt out answers in class without waiting to be called on or hear the whole question.
Intrude on other people's conversations or games.

Often interrupt others; say the wrong thing at the wrong time.

Be unable to keep powerful emotions in check, resulting in angry outbursts or temper tantrums.

Positive effects of ADHD in children

ADHD has nothing to do with intelligence or talent. What's more, kids with attention deficit disorder often demonstrate the following positive traits:

Creativity. Children who have ADHD can be marvelously creative and imaginative. The child who daydreams and has ten different thoughts at once can become a master problem-solver, a fountain of ideas, or an inventive artist. Children with ADHD may be easily distracted, but sometimes they notice what others don't see.

Flexibility. Because children with ADHD consider a lot of options at once, they don't become set on one alternative early on and are more open to different ideas.

Enthusiasm and spontaneity. Children with ADHD are rarely boring! They're interested in a lot of different things and have lively personalities. In short, if they're not exasperating you (and sometimes even when they are), they're a lot of fun to be with.

Energy and drive. When kids with ADHD are motivated, they work or play hard and strive to succeed. It actually may be difficult to distract them from a task that interests them, especially if the activity is interactive or hands-on.

Is it really ADHD?
Just because a child has symptoms of inattention, impulsivity, or hyperactivity does not mean that they have ADHD. Certain medical conditions, psychological disorders, and stressful life events can cause symptoms that look like ADHD.

Before an accurate diagnosis of ADHD can be made, it is important that you see a mental health professional to explore and rule out the following possibilities:

Learning disabilities or problems with reading, writing, motor skills, or language.

Major life events or traumatic experiences, such as a recent move, death of a loved one, bullying, or divorce.

Psychological disorders including anxiety, depression, or bipolar disorder.

Behavioral disorders such as conduct disorder, reactive attachment disorder, and oppositional defiant disorder.

Medical conditions, including thyroid problems, neurological conditions, epilepsy, and sleep disorders.

Helping a child with ADHD

Whether or not your child's symptoms of inattention, hyperactivity, and impulsivity are due to ADHD, they can cause many problems if left untreated. Children who can't focus and control themselves may struggle in school, get into frequent trouble, and find it hard to get along with others or make friends. These frustrations and difficulties can lead to low self-esteem as well as friction and stress for the whole family.

But treatment can make a dramatic difference in your child's symptoms. With the right support, your child can get on track for success in all areas of life.

If your child struggles with symptoms that look like ADHD, don't wait to seek professional help. You can treat your child's symptoms of hyperactivity, inattention, and impulsivity without having a diagnosis of attention deficit disorder. Options to start with include getting your child into therapy, implementing a better diet and exercise plan, and modifying the home environment to minimize distractions.

If you do receive a diagnosis of ADHD, you can then work with your child's doctor, therapist, and school to make a personalized treatment plan that meets their specific needs. Effective treatment for childhood ADHD involves behavioral therapy, parent education and training, social support, and assistance at school. Medication may also be used; however, it should never be the sole attention deficit disorder treatment.

Parenting tips for children with ADHD
If your child is hyperactive, inattentive, or impulsive, it may take a lot of energy to get them to listen, finish a task, or sit still. The constant monitoring can be frustrating and exhausting. Sometimes you may feel like your child is running the show. But there are steps you can take to regain control of the

situation, while simultaneously helping your child make the most of their abilities.

While attention deficit disorder is not caused by bad parenting, there are effective parenting strategies that can go a long way to correct problem behaviors. Children with ADHD need structure, consistency, clear communication, and rewards and consequences for their behavior. They also need lots of love, support, and encouragement.

There are many things parents can do to reduce the signs and symptoms of ADHD without sacrificing the natural energy, playfulness, and sense of wonder unique in every child.

Take care of yourself so you're better able to care for your child. Eat right, exercise, get enough sleep, find ways to reduce stress, and seek face-to-face support from family and friends as well as your child's doctor and teachers.

Establish structure and stick to it. Help your child stay focused and organized by following daily routines, simplifying your child's schedule, and keeping your child busy with healthy activities.

Set clear expectations. Make the rules of behavior simple and explain what will happen when they are obeyed or broken—and follow through each time with a reward or a consequence.

Encourage exercise and sleep. Physical activity improves concentration and promotes brain growth. Importantly for children with ADHD, it also leads to better sleep, which in turn can reduce the symptoms of ADHD.

Help your child eat right. To manage symptoms of ADHD, schedule regular healthy meals or snacks every three hours and cut back on junk and sugary food.

Teach your child how to make friends. Help them become a better listener, learn to read people's faces and body language, and interact more smoothly with others.

School tips for children with ADHD
ADHD, obviously, gets in the way of learning. You can't absorb information or get your work done if you're running around the classroom or zoning out on what you're supposed to be reading or listening to. Think of what the school setting requires children to do: Sit still. Listen quietly. Pay attention. Follow instructions. Concentrate. These are the very things kids with ADHD have a hard time doing—not because they aren't willing, but because their brains won't let them.

But that doesn't mean kids with ADHD can't succeed at school. There are many things both parents and teachers can do to help children with ADHD thrive in the classroom. It starts with evaluating each child's individual weaknesses and strengths, then coming up with creative strategies for helping them focus, stay on task, and learn to their full capability.

CHAPTER 3

HOW TO IDENTIFY PARENTING TRIGGERS AND 10 WAYS TO DEAL WITH THEM

Does it feel like you are always yelling at your child? Tired of being calm at one moment and angry at the next? Why couldn't he listen the first time? Or why are they always fighting and screaming? Or only if she just stops throwing all her toys, I wouldn't have to get angry. " Tons of techniques to control your child's behaviour can help you, but if you are unable to control your behaviour, that will be a bigger issue.

Instead of focusing on your kid's behaviour, let's have a look at what's bothering you.
When I thought of becoming a parent, I thought I must have understood this parenting thing thoroughly. I thought that I would be the most patient, calm, loving

mama who took it all in her stride and responded with compassion and empathy to her kids. If you're anything like me, you would have imagined what becoming a parent would be like: taking trips to parks, arts and crafts projects, pretend plays, bedtime stories, and things like that. Parenting triggers are not something you gave a thought about before becoming a parent, right? Sure, you knew that there would be difficulties and struggles, but you always pictured how you would handle them patiently and calmly.

What you might not have imagined was losing it when the toddler refuses to eat the food that you've lovingly prepared for them, the whining that starts just before you thought of relaxing while having a hot cup of coffee for yourself and a book to read, or siblings fighting over the TV remote to watch their favourite shows. Every parent has a skeleton in their parenting closet. We all get triggered! We all react, yell, shame, spank, and whatnot. We all get into situations where it just gets to us and we react in ways we never expected to behave.

Those are the toughest moments of our parenting journey where we start doubting ourselves as parents. These reactions to triggers challenge our self-perception and create a mismatch between what we believe as parents and how we behave, making the parenting journey more difficult. So here are 10 ways to identify parenting triggers and how to deal with them.

What are the parenting triggers?

Parenting Triggers are the ones that are caused by our child's behaviour. Sometimes, when they say, do, or feel something and we have an automatic negative response in return, we yell, lash out, shut down, cry, try to escape, or sometimes you feel compelled to punish or shame your children when feel triggered. We may say or do things that we normally wouldn't and feel guilty about it later.

A trigger can be anything when you experience the present moment that activates the feeling from the past. We may act in a way that's not in keeping with the present. A trigger often activates an old wound from our childhood, like not being heard, respected, or taken for granted. Many times, when our children get upset, we get angry or annoyed by their way of expressing certain feelings (whining, tantrums, or crying). It's more often about ourselves than our difficulties in processing these emotions than the child's behaviour.

Triggers cause us to act in a certain way that, as parents, we do not value and believe. Our responses when triggered are usually extreme, and we feel lost, angry, and out of control. They are almost automatic and sometimes out of proportion too, and it is hard to understand why. They are often related to the experiences we get from our childhood, upbringing, or schooling.

Triggers don't always have to be something negative. Our children have done it too. Sometimes it can be a positive experience our child is having that we have never had a chance to trigger in us. Many of us were not "allowed" freedom or independence. We were never free from unnecessary control. So sometimes our children's living this way can trigger us.

The most important part of parenting with a trigger is that you are not reacting to your child's certain ways of behaving, but you are having a reaction because of what that behaviour means to you and that is triggered by your past experiences.

What does a parenting trigger look like?
We all have different triggers, but our children experiencing strong emotions is a huge trigger for many of us. It is often because we were raised in an environment where we were not free to express our emotions safely. If we do so, then it would lead to us being punished, shamed, ignored, or otherwise invalidated. So, when our children go through those emotions, we often feel threatened or overwhelmed by them, or simply do not know how to deal with them because no one ever modelled them for us as children. Even children being "silly" can sometimes bring us back to our inner child who was shamed for being silly. Emotions can be very powerful as a trigger. But I can assure you that this gets easier with time and support.

For many of us, it was punishable to disobey as a child, so when our children do, we often feel confronted and challenged. And it invokes a reactionary response based on what happened to us. Sometimes we get triggered because the things our children do are the things we would have been punished, belittled, shamed, or bullied for. We feel protective and fear they will experience the same things. We have to keep reminding ourselves that our job isn't to stop them from being themselves, but rather to show them that they are unconditionally loved and appreciated for being their authentic selves. We should not unintentionally recreate our fears by stopping them from being themselves. We should advocate for them when people around them aren't respectful.

In some cases, we are triggered when we do not know what to do in that situation because we are not parenting as we are trying to parent, and situations like these can make us feel like it's a lot. I know when I sometimes have moments like these when my daughter is struggling and I do not know what to do to help her and I get triggered into feeling worthless and helpless.

Triggers are as varied as we are as parents. Here are some common parenting triggers that I have heard and experienced:

- Concerns about wasting food.

- Concerns about a child not eating enough and worried about health.

- Concerns about child's safety.

- When children are being authentically themselves.

- Children crying.

- When children don't share.

- Child is unkind.

- Children being dishonest.

- Children are not using manners.

- When Children talk back.

- Children being picky.

- Children being "bossy".

- Behaving rudely.

- Being angry.

- Children throwing a tantrum.

- Children being silly.

- Child not listening to you.

- Child not taking you seriously.

- Loud Noises.

- Mess

- Lack of privacy.

- Lack of personal space.

- Feeling unappreciated.

- Feeling ignored.

- Feeling unheard.

- Feeling touched out.

- Feeling disrespected.

- Feeling tired.

- Feeling overwhelmed.

Many of these are related to feelings and emotions that cause triggers. These triggers can steal the moment from being able to be the parent you want to be. We act impulsively in a protective way to stop our emotional discomfort instead of what we genuinely want for our child.

Some of these things help us respectfully teach our children to navigate their emotions. Many of the time, children deserve to be able to do things that can trigger some emotions in us, but in those instances, we need to parent through these triggers.

Why Is Recognizing Your Triggers Important?

Many of the experts say that there is unresolved trauma that can be passed through generations and continue to plague our kids for a long time. Once you are aware of your triggers, you increase the chances of favouring a positive response to your child's behaviour. What if there are some areas where your unintended, irrational reactions are damaging your child? Then you can start working to resolve these situations. Most of the time, you need to take a step back and analyse the situation before reacting. It will only help you recognize your triggers, and you will react more proactively.

If you start taking significant steps to identify your parenting triggers, you will uncover the roots of your past emotional wounds that are affecting your and your child's relationship. If you understand your triggering points, then you will be able to create a safe and nurturing environment for your child.

How to Identify Your Parenting Triggers?
We all have our own demons, that's for sure. But once you start your journey of getting to know and understanding your triggers, you truly start healing, emotionally and mentally. The key factor in identifying your parenting triggers is to pay attention to your

feelings and look for patterns in your reactions.

The 7 clues to identifying parenting triggers are:

Whenever you feel extremely angry, like yelling, seeing red, or vein pooping, that means you have been triggered.

When you feel sad, upset, or hurt after something your child has said or done to you (that you shouldn't take personally), it means you have been triggered.

If you are upset, angry or fearful, just out of proportion, which you realise once you are calm, you've probably been triggered.

Any time you feel like everything is out of control, you are triggered.

If you feel like you have experienced this kind of feeling many times before and it feels similar, it means you have certainly been triggered.

If you were calm a minute ago and suddenly feel uncontrollable anger inside, you've been triggered.

If you find yourself suddenly wanting to grab, punish, spank, or physically hurt your child, you have been triggered.

How do we deal with parenting triggers?
1.	Ask Yourself: Why am I getting triggered?

If you are reacting aggressively, taking things personally in a situation, then it means you are not reacting towards the situation happening in front of you, but you might be reacting to something that has happened in the past and has been evoked.

When you feel such emotions triggering, start meditation and pay attention to the sensations, visual images, words, or thoughts to decipher the real meaning behind these parenting triggers. These things will help you to understand where you are coming from and how to work on them.

2.   Start Working on It.

Once you are aware of your past hurts and emotional baggage that is currently affecting your reaction to your child, it's time to work on it. Keep a list of the situations when you responded aggressively; they could be a possible trigger. This will help you understand the events better, and you can process them thoroughly once you are calm.

Factors that may have caused anxiety, anger, stress, or insecurity can be re-understood. Working on your past experiences and letting them go and moving on is a huge step.

3.   Change is for the better.

Since you have understood and identified your parenting triggers, it's now time to work on the change. First thing first, start imaging the probable outcomes of the situations that can be different. Focus on how these different responses make you feel. Be aware of your body language, the tone of your voice, and the words you are using while in the situation.

4.   Start small.

You don't need to go all in to change yourself. Start with small changes. Doing it all at once will overwhelm you and it will be hard to tackle. You can start with one thing at a time, such as: what can be done differently next time the situation arises?

Focus on the unmet needs. Our needs being met should not affect our relationship with our children.

5.   Work on Healing.

You need to let go of the shame and guilt caused by the trigger to start healing. Blaming yourself for your actions is not going to do any good to you or your child. Instead, practise self-compassion and empathy. You need to remind yourself that these are the things that will challenge you and that they are perfect learning and growth opportunities for you.

You need to at least try to be kind to yourself as you are to your children. Because you need this kindness to grow as a parent. Empathizing with ourselves does not mean not holding ourselves to high standards and aiming for growth, but it means recognising that what we are doing is hard work and it matters. You need to focus on your improvement and what your child deserves.

6.   Take your time.

Whenever you find yourself in a situation where you feel triggered, take a moment to slow down and relax. Sometimes we feel parenting is urgent, but almost always it is not. You can simply be honest and say, "I am finding it hard; can I take a minute please?"

Taking a step back and giving yourself some space to breathe will help you handle the situation more calmly. Being gentle with yourself and granting some space will help you process the triggers. I know it will be hard to accept and change yourself, but believe me, it's all worth it.

7.   Accept your mistakes and apologise to your child.

Another impactful thing you can do while working on your triggers is to be honest with your children about them. You don't have to give much detail about your triggers to them, but letting our children know about our struggles with finding certain things difficult and that it's not their fault is helpful. This helps them with empathy as well as keeps them in the loop when you are dealing with parenting triggers and you need some space or time to process them.

Also, having a parental tantrum gives you the perfect opportunity to teach your child the art of a well-formed apology. You need to make it sincere and direct. Take full responsibility for your behaviour and make it clear to them that you will take active steps to work on your behaviour in the future. You can say something like, "Hey, I am sorry for yelling at you like that when you spilt the milk. I was overreacting and I am sure I made you feel horrible. It is hard for me to handle the mess. Still, it was not OK for me to yell like that, and I am going to work on remaining calm and talking more constructively in the future. "

8.   Understand childhood development.

It is important to be aware of your child's development at a given age to know what is reasonable and appropriate to expect from them. Being aware of the information will help you adjust your expectations and prepare you for the behaviours that might trigger-induce you.

9.   Seek help.

If you find yourself consistently angry and have trouble controlling it, then finding a mental health professional may be the most important option for you. You can't always manage or change things on your own. Triggers from your past relationships, childhood trauma, anxiety, or depression can be too difficult to change without support.

10. Surround yourself with support.

Having like-minded and supportive friends who are themselves parents is essential in the parenting journey. Being surrounded by people who understand and who encourage you in this process is very helpful. Some might become nurturing figures for us. It is important to not feel alone on this journey and to have people who value what you are doing and value children the way you do. We aren't supposed to do this alone, and having a network that shares this lifestyle is very powerful.

With time, you will be able to analyse your triggering situations and be able to intervene before you react with anger.

Even if you do get triggered, all is not lost! Give yourself some time out, take a deep breath, and think it through.

Remember, parenting is all about learning and growing. The more you learn, the better choices you will make next time!

FAQs

1.   What drives people angry?

There are several common triggers for anger, such as losing patience, feeling like your efforts are not appreciated, or injustice towards you. Also, childhood traumas or abuse, extreme anxiety, or depression can cause anger in people.

2.   What does "triggered" mean?

Triggers are anything that reminds someone of their past traumatic experiences. For example, visual images of violence can be a trigger point for some people. Sometimes, for someone, odours, perfumes, songs, or even colours can be triggers, depending upon their past experiences.

3.   What is the trigger behaviour?

When someone reacts in anger towards a particular situation, it is often called "trigger behaviour". This kind of behaviour is usually preceded and caused by a violent outburst. They are often verbal or non-verbal behaviours that bring up a feeling of abandonment and rejection.

4.   How do you identify a trigger in a child?
To identify triggers in a child, you need to discuss and label the physical feelings that are associated with triggers. After a tantrum or meltdown, talk with your child about the feelings they feel in their body. Discuss things like racing heartbeats, hot red faces, and lumps in the throat that indicate your child's anger is escalating. These practices

will help you analyse if your child has been triggered.

CHAPTER 4

BEEN A COMPASSIONATE PARENT

Compassion is a central aspect of the human condition. It refers to the ability to be present to our suffering and that of others without ignoring it, minimising it, judging it, or running away from it, and responding with a desire to relieve this suffering with an attitude of kindness, care, and support.

Being compassionate has been linked to increased well-being and it is no different when it comes to parenting. It has been shown that compassionate parenting promotes better parent-child relationships (Duncan, Coatsworth & Greenberg, 2009), which in turn helps our children to grow up feeling more secure, connected, and ultimately more compassionate themselves.

So, how can parents show compassion in their daily interactions with their children?

1. Generate a safe space
Parents' primary responsibility is to foster a safe space where the child feels able to communicate freely and openly. You may begin by inviting your child to share their feelings. And when they start to open up, just listen. Make sure the child is not interrupted or criticised but be listened to non-judgmentally. This will help to really get to know our children, bond with them, and cherish them.

2. Being a child is not so easy
Remember that there are numerous stressors that children need to manage, such as school pressures, getting good grades, making friends, emotional and physical changes, social media, amongst others. Yet, they are expected to manage all these stressors despite lacking in life experience to guide them. So, the next time your child gets

upset about "little things", see if you can understand the situation from their perspective. What might seem trivial to a parent, might mean a lot to the child.

3. Parent to prepare
Despite our good intentions, when we try to protect our children from experiencing failure, we are holding them back from developing the skills needed to tolerate their difficult experiences and do what is needed to relieve their suffering. For example, failing an exam does not need to be portrayed as a catastrophe. Instead, validate and allow yourself to be present with your child's feelings by saying something like "It's disappointing when you don't pass an exam" and encouraging them to try to make up for it in the next exam.

4. Believe your child has the capability to be compassionate
The beliefs that children develop about themselves are very much influenced by

their parents' beliefs about them. For instance, if the child is branded as a troublemaker, it is likely his behaviour will eventually end up reflecting that belief. Conversely, if we believe the child is capable of being compassionate, this can help us respond to them more compassionately without criticism, blame, or shame, thus fostering the belief that the child is worthy of compassion. In other words, what we believe about our children goes a very long way!

5. Be compassionate to yourself when setbacks happen
Parenting is hard work and there are many challenges that parents face daily. In order to be compassionate towards your children, you need to first learn to give compassion to yourself. You may do this by first noticing when you are being hard on yourself (e.g., "I'm such a bad parent"), remind yourself that raising children is an important and difficult job, and finally offer something

kind to yourself, such as "Parenting is hard
and I'm not alone in this".

CHAPTER 5

LISTENING TO YOUR KIDS (8 Reasons to Listen to Your Child | Positive Parenting)

I admit that I am a pretty ordinary listener.

You see by nature I am a talker and a fixer. Tell me a problem and I want to talk it through and find the best answer for with you. It's just how I am. Lately however I have had to work on stifling my first reaction – to talk and solve – and learn to do a better job of listening, of giving Immy especially space and time to talk and find her own answers. Which is not always easy for a fixer like me.

And it's not only the fixing that can be the problem. There's the busyness of everyday life and the myriad of demands on my time and attention and the distractions of technology, just to name a few. All this means that at times it is way too easy to be remote and distracted, or sometimes even offhandedly dismissive of my children's efforts to engage me.

But I know that it is important to listen. To listen without fixing. To listen without judgment. To listen until small people have had plenty of time to form and articulate their thoughts.

To be fully present and listen.

So I have been working hard to remind myself why it's important. Here are eight reasons I have come up with...

Reason #1: It strengthens the parent-child bond.
My Mum is still one of the first people I turn to when I need a shoulder to cry on or someone to vent to. I can go to her with ideas or problems or news or just to chat about the mundane of everyday and I know

she will listen. I want my children to have that same feeling that they can come to me with anything at all and I will listen and be there for them.

To be truly heard is to know that our thoughts and feelings, dreams and fears can be expressed and known; that who we really are has a place in this world. - Gerry Fewster

Reason #2: It opens the lines of communication. And you want them open.
I think in many ways we are still in the easy years of communication with our young family (yes, even with a toddler in the early verbal stage of development). I expect that it is when my girls hit the tween and teen years that this reason will become even more important to our relationship. I want to know what is going on in their lives – the good and the bad.

Tip: If technology is distracting you from being present with your children, commit to regular technology-free time. Leave the computer or phone off until they are busy with other things or in bed.

Reason #3: It improves the likelihood that they will in turn listen to you.
When a person feels respected and appreciated, they are much more likely to respond in turn with respect and appreciation. And in this way, children are no different to adults. Connection is so vitally important to influence.

Reason #4: It helps to build self esteem.
Your time and your attention are valuable, kids know that, and by giving them your undivided time and attention they feel valued which is great for their developing self esteem.

"Be who you are and say what you feel because those who mind don't matter and those who matter don't mind." Dr Seuss

Tip: Try to build regular one-on-one time with each of your children into your week. Immy has recently started joining me as I walk/jog for exercise on the weekends. We are both really enjoying this time together – in fact, just last weekend she chose walking with me over watching something on TV. Those that know her well know that my girl loves her TV time so this was kind of a big deal.

Reason #5: It helps them to feel understood. It is important to listen with the intent to understand, not to reply (or to fix!) Asking a specific question in response to what they say lets your child know you are really listening, validates what they are telling you and hopefully keeps the conversation going.

"Most people do not listen with the intent to understand; they listen with the intent to reply." Stephen R Covey
Reason #6: It provides insight into their emotional state.

I was fascinated to read the research shared by Michael Grose about the connection between regular family conversation and anxiety and depressive illnesses in young people;

"The biggest single preventative factor for anxiety and depressive illnesses in young people is being in a family that has 5-6 shared meals together with the television and other communication devices off." Read more here.

Tip: Eat together as a family as regularly as you can – remember it isn't just dinner that counts.

Reason #7: It helps them to develop effective social skills.
Your attentive listening provides your child with a fabulous role model for the development of positive social relationships. They learn about the give and take of

conversation and how good it feels to be heard.

Reason #8: Because kids have great ideas. Children have great ideas and it is through talking through these ideas that many people (children included) are able to plan a course of action and make these ideas come to fruition.

Tip: Make some of your everyday travel time technology free for everyone, especially if you are travelling with just one of your kids.

CHAPTER 6

HANDLING DIFFICULT FEELINGS (7 Steps to Manage Difficult Emotions)

It might seem counterintuitive but facing your emotions can support you in processing them.
Written by Jerusha Kamoji, expert review by Rebecca Acabchuk, Ph.D.
7 Steps to Manage Difficult Emotions
"Negative thoughts, emotions, and beliefs are said to be like Velcro; they stick easier than their positive counterparts," says Rebecca Acabchuk, Ph.D., a neuroscientist and senior researcher at Roundglass. While it's normal to have a negativity bias, getting stuck on it can lead to unnecessary suffering because you may create more of what you don't want to experience.

According to David Vago, Ph.D., Roundglass research lead and neuroscientist, some recent scientific reviews suggest focusing on depressive thoughts and negative emotions, like anger and fear, can increase the wear and tear on your body, therefore accelerate aging.

"The evidence even supports that if these types of thoughts and emotions are not properly managed, they can lead to pervasive inflammation contributing significantly to neurodegenerative disorders like Alzheimer's and Parkinson's disease," he says. Over time, persistent negative thoughts and emotions can weaken your immune response, making you more susceptible to developing diseases.

This doesn't mean you should suppress negative feelings either, as research suggests that ignoring them can harm your physical health. It might seem counterintuitive but facing your emotions can support you in processing them.

Use Emotional Awareness to Manage Difficult Emotions
Being emotionally aware means you notice your feelings, name them, and allow yourself to experience their rise and fall. It's a balance between releasing the need to control their intensity and not letting them consume you.

Connecting to your breath while witnessing your feelings can support you in learning about your triggers. It's also a great way to learn that emotions aren't permanent.

Pro Tip: "You can recognize their [emotions] impermanence while learning what may have caused them to arise," says Kasandra Jewall, a Roundglass yoga teacher.

Use Emotional Awareness to See the Temporary Nature of Emotions
When you allow yourself to be emotionally aware, you learn to recognize emotions for

what they are — simple sensory experiences passing through your awareness.

You can think of this awareness like an emotional digestive system. But, instead of breaking down the foods you eat and absorbing their nutrients into your cells and bloodstream, you're absorbing and processing your experiences.

It can be hard to control the things or people who might trigger your emotions, but channeling that energy into digesting these experiences makes managing difficult emotions that much easier. "Your ability to understand yourself and why you feel the way you feel will give you a more grounded space to react from," Jewall says.

Here are 7 mindfulness-infused tips that can support you as you learn to digest difficult emotions.

Managing Difficult Emotions: A Mindful Practice

1. Invite In What Is

Dr. Acabchuk suggests rather than viewing emotions as good or bad, try allowing yourself to become curious about how you feel, without any judgment toward the feelings themselves.

Pro Tip: "Ask yourself, 'How am I feeling today?' and welcome all that arises, with an honest, open heart," Dr. Acabchuk says.

2. Recognize and Name Your Feeling(s)

Naming your feeling can help you step back and look at it from a distance. This separation creates space for you to calm your body and settle your mind.

This labeling practice has other benefits, too. "Increased emotion identification is related to higher levels of perceived control, fewer negative thoughts, and healthier relationships," Dr. Vago says.

Pro Tip: The Roundglass Feelings Wheel can help you label your emotions more specifically, leading to greater insight. At the center of the wheel are seven primary emotions and the two larger circles include a variety of feelings. "Emotions are the automatic responses that appear before certain stimuli, such as the sadness we experience when we lose a loved one," Dr. Acabchuk says. "Feelings are the subjective perceptions of emotions, the way each of us interprets the emotion and gives it a name."

3. Accept the Emotion as Part of Your Present Experience

Trying to push difficult feelings away doesn't make them disappear. Buried emotions can leak out at times, especially under stress, causing you to act in ways that you might regret later.

This could look like speaking to colleagues in a short manner or raising your voice to your kids when you don't mean to. Use meditation to accept the existence of difficult emotions, which allows you to experience and then release them.

4. Assure Yourself the Emotion Is a Phase

"My silent retreat meditation practice helped me understand that every emotion has a beginning, a middle, and an end," says Grace Edmunds, a Roundglass meditation teacher.

Recognizing the impermanence of your emotions can help you witness them without feeling overwhelmed or personalizing them. Reminding yourself, "this too shall pass," can provide strength to endure challenging times.

Try this class, Find Emotional Balance, by Dr. David Vago to learn how to embrace the impermanence of your emotions.

5. Understand the Emotion

When you know what you feel, you can learn why you feel, and knowing this may help you better process the experience. Toni Parker, Ph.D., a certified Gottman therapist, suggests asking yourself questions like, "what triggered me?" Or "why do I feel this way?" after you've calmed down.

"Asking yourself these critical questions and investigating the root of your difficult emotions will help you gain empathy and insight into what you are experiencing," she writes.

Try this class, Embrace Your Emotions, by Greta Hill, a Roundglass meditation teacher, to learn how to objectively experience your emotions so you can understand them.

6. Let Go of the Need to Control Your Emotional State

It's normal to want to control your emotions, especially when they seem overwhelming. However, Jewall recommends doing something active the next time you feel the need to suppress those intense feelings. Moving your body can support you in processing what she calls "emotional energy."

"I would encourage people to do meditation or something active like yoga to help them move emotional energy," she says. If you can't move your body, Jewall recommends drawing. "Even taking a piece of paper and scribbling may bring insight," she adds.

One study found that young, middle-aged, and older adults who engaged in high and moderate levels of exercise had higher life satisfaction than the participants who engaged in low levels of exercise. This means they were more likely to experience positive emotions when they thought about the unique circumstances of their lives. Positive thinking and positive emotions can make it easier to experience and recover from stress.

7. Identify and Embrace Emotional Suffering

Pain is universal; something we all sense, yet we often feel alone in times of distress.

Reminding yourself that everyone experiences pain, and that suffering is part of the human condition can bring comfort during times of adversity. And Metta or loving-kindness meditations can help you nurture this knowledge. One part of the practice asks you to recognize shared humanity by telling yourself, "I'm not the only one suffering in this way."

Taking this broader view can shift your attention away from yourself, to help avoid developing a victim mindset. "By reprogramming the way, we think, and what we focus our attention on, we can transform the way we feel and how we live our lives," Dr. Vago says.

Learning to manage difficult emotions takes repetition and focus. But honouring the existence of challenging feelings can help you find unique ways to process them. In addition to the 7 mindful coping strategies, a complementary practice includes finding the positive.

Practicing positive thinking can make a big difference when it comes to managing emotional workloads.

Use These 7 Steps to Practice Positive Thinking

Humans have an ingrained negativity bias because it helps to protect us from harm, "remember the threat, to help you remain safe," Dr. Acabchuk says. It's why you tend to recall, then focus on, one piece of negative feedback in a presentation that went well.

However, it's important to practice positive thinking because it can increase resilience to stress. "Some stressors are unavoidable, but we do have some power over how our thoughts and emotions contribute to our mental and physical health." Dr. Vago says.

Instead of focusing on feeling anxious about being late while sitting in a traffic jam, use mindfulness to notice that you're anxious. Then practice positive thinking by being grateful for having a car or getting some extra time to listen to music.

Simply being aware of what you tell yourself can help you pause and choose to find the positive.

Pro Tip: "Gratitude, compassion, awe, and curiosity are all techniques that strengthen positive thinking," Dr. Acabchuck says.

While everyone's emotional experience is unique, infusing mindfulness as you practice positive thinking can support you in feeling and healing whatever difficult emotion you're facing. Here are some examples.

Soothe Sadness
With social stereotypes and gender norms, sadness might be one of the most difficult emotions to express. But to soothe sadness, you'll have to feel it. This could look like bellowing into a pillow, replaying your favorite Adele album, or simply sitting and being with your sadness. However, you choose to express it, remember that sadness

is just an emotion, and it will, like all emotions, pass.

Sadness is different from depression because of its temporary nature. Depression can happen when you've lost interest in all the things that used to bring you joy. You may also find you spend more time alone, not because it's rejuvenating, but because you feel isolated.

Pro Tip: If you're experiencing depression, try seeking professional help, as it's considered a "mental illness and should be treated seriously," Dr. Vago says.

Unpack Shame
Many people may use guilt and shame interchangeably, but shame researcher Brené Brown separates the two. Shame focuses on the self, and guilt focuses on the action. You can think of shame as saying, "I am embarrassing," versus guilt; "I did something embarrassing." While both

feelings are harmful, shame can be more dangerous because "it can chip away at our self-worth," Dr. Vago says.

Outside of meditation, Dr. Vago recommends finding a safe environment where you can openly talk about your feelings of shame. "If there was shame for a specific behavior, it would be typical to speak to a psychologist or supportive group therapy to unpack the shame and associated clinical symptoms," he says. This is because shame is usually tied to having some secret, and letting it out can help you understand and release it.

Pro Tip: "Seeking out a supportive environment to discuss feelings of shame can help them dissipate," Dr. Vago says.

Dial Down Fear
"Being scared and experiencing fear are two of the same expressions of one of the most primal universal emotions," Dr. Acabchuk

says. Fear also varies in intensity; you may experience nervousness or uneasiness on the low end, and panic or horror if you're very scared.

Fear isn't always bad because it can help prepare you for potential threats. It can, however, become destabilizing if the threat is perceived as overwhelming. "We may experience helplessness, further anxiety, and thoughts that prolong the stress response," Dr. Vago says.

This can also lead to developing a phobia — a persistent irrational fear.

To dial down fear, try to calm your nervous system through deep breathing. Remind yourself that it's just your body trying to protect itself, and this feeling will pass.

Pro Tip: If you're dealing with a phobia, seek mindfulness-informed, exposure therapy from a trained individual. "Learning how to breathe through the waves of emotion can support dealing with phobias," Dr. Acabchuk says.

Defuse Anger
Analytical anger meditations can help you understand and calm your anger. The practice invites you to consider a series of questions that include, "how is this anger affecting other people and me?" Or "where am I holding that anger in my body?"

Answering these questions may help you recognize your triggers. Knowing this can support you in setting a specific remedy for each.

It can be dangerous to suppress anger, but it also shouldn't be let out by reacting to your trigger at that moment. This is because you're likely teaching your brain to habituate a pattern of exploding when angry.

Whenever you feel enraged, ground down to your breath as you remember that antidote you've set for yourself during meditation. Whether taking a walk, splashing cold water on your face, or simply connecting to the pause between each breath, allow yourself to feel the anger so you can mindfully respond and release it.

Pro Tip: Practice the analytical anger meditations when you're calm for greater insight into your triggers and more clarity to develop antidotes.

Cope with Grief and Loss
You might be mourning the loss of a loved one or drastic changes in your relationship(s), health, or life. The uncertainty, rage, and despair that come with that may sometimes feel as if you want to implode. But connecting with other people who are suffering in the same way may help.

In one study, caregivers experiencing grief for the death of cancer patients they nursed found sharing their stories of suffering helped to make them feel less alone and less stressed. They also found it easier to make sense of their situations.

Dr. Vago recommends grief counseling if you find you are struggling to recover from the loss of a loved one. It may offer a more personalized approach in helping you cope with the intensity of your emotions, which you can use long after you decide to stop going.

Pro Tip: If you're interested in seeing a grief counselor, try going to one that includes body scans or other mindfulness meditation practices, as they may "help to restore a sense of ease in the body," Dr. Vago says.

Learn to Ride the Waves of Your Emotions
When you think of difficult emotions, Jewall suggests imagining your mind as a ship

drifting through them. Like waves, they come and go; like waves, they can wreck you. But you can always use emotional awareness as a sail to "catch and harnesses mindful practices" that can help you identify, experience, and better manage your difficult emotions.

CHAPTER 7

UTTERING APPROPRIATE WORDS/POSITIVE THINGS TO SAY TO KIDS: ENCOURAGING WORDS FOR KIDS

Research has been done to show that the kind of praise that we give to our children can ultimately influence them and motivate them later in life. Therefore, when we utter these words of encouragement to our children, we want to focus on the effort rather than their talent.

The best thing you can do is show them encouragement when they try their best. It doesn't matter if their abilities are top-notch or above others; they are looking for encouragement at that moment as they put their effort into the task at hand.

Choosing specific phrases to use can also help encourage them. Don't generalize your words of encouragement too much. Be specific to what they are working to accomplish. If they are painting a picture, for example, focus on the different colors they have chosen rather than just saying good job.

You also want to be careful to avoid giving them TOO MUCH praise. Too much praise can actually result in negative effects down the line. They will begin to think that they no longer have to try to succeed and their self-confidence may be off the charts. Remember, as parents; we are looking to encourage them while making a positive impact.

The praise you offer your children should also be sincere and honest. If the praise you are offering doesn't feel sincere, then they will likely not feel encouraged at all. The praise is ultimately discounted and can lead to a child to practice self-criticism.

CHAPTER 8

ATTENTIVE PROBLEM-SOLVING

Problem-solving is an important life skill for teenagers.

You can help teenagers learn to solve problems by working through our 6 steps together.

Calm communication, active listening and compromise are also important in problem-solving.

Problem-solving: 6 steps
1. Identify the problem
2. Think about why it's a problem
3. Brainstorm possible solutions to the problem
4. Evaluate the solutions to the problem
5. Put the solution into action
6. Evaluate the outcome of your problem-solving process
Why problem-solving skills are important

Everybody needs to solve problems every day. But we're not born with the skills we need to do this – we have to develop them.

When you're solving problems, it's good to be able to:

listen and think calmly
consider options and respect other people's opinions and needs
negotiate and work towards compromises.
These are skills for life – they're highly valued in both social and work situations.

When teenagers learn skills and strategies for problem-solving and sorting out conflicts by themselves, they feel good about themselves. They're better placed to make good decisions on their own.

Problem-solving: 6 steps
Often you can solve problems by talking and negotiating.

The following 6 steps for problem-solving are useful when you can't find a solution. You can use them to work on most problems, including difficult choices or decisions and conflicts between people.

If you practise these steps with your child at home, your child is more likely to use them with their own problems or conflicts with others.

You might like to download and use our problem-solving worksheet (PDF: 121kb). It's a handy tool to use as you and your child work together through the 6 steps below.

1. Identify the problem
The first step in problem-solving is working out exactly what the problem is. This can help everyone understand the problem in the same way. It's best to get everyone who's affected by the problem together and then put the problem into words that make it solvable.

For example:

'You've been invited to two birthday parties on the same day and you want to go to both.'
'You have two big assignments due next Wednesday.'
'We have different ideas about how you'll get home from the party on Saturday.'
'You and your sister have been arguing about using the Xbox.'
When you're working on a problem with your child, it's good to do it when everyone is calm and can think clearly. This way, your child will be more likely to want to find a solution. Arrange a time when you won't be interrupted, and thank your child for joining in to solve the problem.

2. Think about why it's a problem
Help your child or children describe what's causing the problem and where it's coming from. It might help to consider answers to questions like these:

Why is this so important to you?
Why do you need this?
What do you think might happen?
What's upsetting you?
What's the worst thing that could happen?
Try to listen without arguing or debating. This is your chance to really hear what's going on with your child. Encourage your child to use statements like 'I need … I want … I feel …', and try using these phrases yourself. Try to encourage your child to focus on the issue and keep blame out of this step.

Some conflict is natural and healthy, but too much isn't a good thing. If you find you're clashing with your child a lot, you can use conflict management strategies. This can make future conflict less likely, and it's good for your family relationships too.

3. Brainstorm possible solutions to the problem

Make a list of all the possible ways you and your child could solve the problem. You're looking for a range of possibilities, both sensible and not so sensible. Try to avoid judging or debating these yet.

If your child has trouble coming up with solutions, start them off with some suggestions of your own. You could set the tone by making a crazy suggestion first – funny or extreme solutions can end up sparking more helpful options. Try to come up with at least 5 possible solutions together.

For example, if your children are arguing about using the Xbox, here are some possible solutions:

'We buy another Xbox so you don't have to share.'
'The two of you agree on when you can each use the Xbox.'
'You each have set days for using the Xbox.'

'You each get to use the Xbox for 30 minutes a day.'
'You put away the Xbox until next year.'
Write down all your possible solutions.

4. Evaluate the solutions to the problem
Look at the pros and cons of all the suggested solutions in turn. This way, everyone will feel that their suggestions have been considered.

It might help to cross off solutions that you all agree aren't acceptable. For example, you might all agree that leaving your children to agree on sharing the Xbox isn't an option because they've already tried that and it hasn't worked.

When you have a list of pros and cons for the remaining solutions, cross off the ones that have more negatives than positives. Now rate each solution from 0 (not good) to 10 (very good). This will help you sort out the most promising solutions.

The solution you and your child choose should be one that your child can put into practice and that could solve the problem.

If you haven't been able to find one that looks promising, go back to step 3 and look for some different solutions. It might help to talk to other people, like other family members, to get a fresh range of ideas.

Sometimes you might not be able to find a solution that makes everyone happy. But by negotiating and compromising, you should be able to find a solution that everyone can live with.

5. Put the solution into action
Once you've agreed on a solution, plan exactly how it will work. It can help to do this in writing, and to include the following points:

Who will do what?

When will they do it?

What's needed to put the solution into action?

In the Xbox example, the agreed solution is 'You each get to use the Xbox for 30 minutes a day'. Here's how you could plan how the solution will work:

Who will do what? Your children will have turns at different times of the day.

When will they do it? One child will have the first turn after they finish their homework. The other child will have their turn after dinner, when their friends are playing.

What's needed? You need a timer, so each child knows when to stop.

You could also talk about when you'll meet again to look at how the solution is working.

By putting time and energy into developing your child's problem-solving skills, you send the message that you value your child's input into important decisions and you think they're capable of managing their own problems. This is good for your relationship with your child.

6. Evaluate the outcome of your problem-solving process
Once your child or children have put the plan into action, you need to check how it went and help them go through the process again if they need to.

Remember that your child will need to give the solution time to work and that not all solutions will work. Sometimes they'll need to try more than one solution. Part of effective problem-solving is being able to adapt when things don't go as well as expected.

Ask your child the following questions:

What has worked well?
What hasn't worked so well?
What could you or we do differently to make the solution work more smoothly?

If the solution hasn't worked, go back to step 1 of this problem-solving process and start again. Perhaps the problem wasn't what you thought it was, or the solutions weren't quite right.

Problem-solving with teenagers: demonstration

View video transcript

In this short video demonstration, two teenage siblings are having a problem sharing and respecting each other's space. So far, they haven't been able to solve the problem themselves, and this has led to conflict and fights. Their father uses a problem-solving approach to resolve their ongoing conflict.

Try to use these skills and steps when you have your own problems to solve or decisions to make. If your child sees you actively dealing with problems using this approach, they might be more likely to try it themselves.

CHAPTER 9

ASSISTING YOUR PEACEFULl HOME (8
SIMPLE WAYS TO CREATE A PEACEFUL
HOME)

These are certainly challenging times. As we
practice social distancing for our own
well-being as well as for our loved ones and
communities, many find themselves cooped
up inside their homes most days. While
there are of course exceptions like the
occasional visits to grocery stores, these are
not necessarily the most peaceful or relaxing
activities.

Our homes are often a place to unwind,
settle in, and escape after a long day out;
now we find ourselves negotiating the
balance between many concerns,
responsibilities, and trying to keep our
minds calm through it all. Not surprisingly,
our surroundings have such a profound
effect on how we feel day to day.

One way to reinfuse a bit of peace and relaxation into your home is by being intentional about your living space. Creating routines, making a few minor changes to decorations, and keeping your senses happy can make all the difference for your mood. And while we find ourselves inside most days, now is a great opportunity to rethink creating a peaceful home environment.

1. De-clutter where you can

Declutter - How to Create a Peaceful Home and Peaceful Environment

An uncluttered home can truly translate to a more clear and calm state of mind. By tidying up the bedroom or simply cleaning knick-knacks off of the kitchen counter, we give ourselves a way to focus when we are feeling more overwhelmed. With less clutter around us, settling our mind is much easier and within reach. We've all likely experienced less memorable nights where external chaos or a mess subconsciously added to our internal stress. A little organization can go a long way to a peaceful home, especially when there are multiple people sharing one living space.

2. Create routines & rituals

Create routines and rituals - 8 Ways to Create a Peaceful Home and Peaceful Environment

Keeping up with routines like getting dressed for the day, cooking healthy meals and sleeping on time remind us of normalcy and motivates us, which is so important in times of uncertainty. If you're looking for ways to adjust to working from home, creating a ritual of walking in the fresh air, afternoon stretching, or tea breaks may help you refocus. And if you have little ones at home, starting simple routines together throughout the day eases stress and adds comfort during the transition. Of course, new rituals such as taking time to check in on relatives or video chat with friends are important ways to stay connected.

3. Use aromatherapy

Aromatherapy Candles - How to Create a Peaceful Home and Peaceful Environment

Filling a room with one of your favorite essential-oil based scents can give you an immediate a sense of peace. A fresh, sweet or woodsy scent is able to boost your mood and can transport your mind to a soothing place in nature. We love lighting a Happiness Candle in our own home to remind us of the seaside or mountain, or adding a little Harmony inside when we need a moment of relaxation and peaceful environment with a Tranquility Candle.

4. Bring nature inside

Bring nature inside - 8 Ways to Create a Peaceful Home and Peaceful Environment

Besides being a beautiful visual to see and a fresh reminder of spring, indoor plants add a touch of energy and life wherever they are scattered around, whether it is on the coffee table, living room mantle or bedside. On its own, greenery helps purify the air you breathe in while bringing soothing colors. Beyond this, rituals like tending to plants by watering or misting can calm your mind in a peaceful environment. Every newly grown green leaf and flower bud gives a reason to appreciate the little things that continue to spark joy.

5. Be mindful of light

Be mindful of light - How to Create a Peaceful Home and Peaceful Environment

With spring finally here, we have more reasons to open the windows to let in some natural light. While at home, choosing warm light over florescent light has an effect on our state of mind. In the later evenings and on rainy days, lighting a candle or turning on a smaller lamp creates a cozy feeling of comfort that is much welcomed. And after a seemingly endless day of juggling kids and work, making a practice of adding candlelight to the dinner table can soothe the kids as well.

8. Find a sanctuary

Find a sanctuary - 8 Ways to Create a Peaceful Home and Peaceful Environment on the Prosperity Candle blog

Each of us deserves a small place to unwind and de-stress that we can call our own. Whether yours is the bathroom transformed into a makeshift spa, the porch where while it's quiet in the morning, or a cozy knitting nook upstairs, this is where you go to rest your mind and body. In the midst of chaos at home, you can feel peace knowing this retreat is awaiting you whenever you need it most.

7. Designate spaces

Designate Space - How to Create a Peaceful Home and Peaceful Environment

Much like creating a sanctuary, designating a home "office" area can free up your thoughts when you are spending time with loved ones or reflecting. This small practice makes work/life balance easier to manage, especially in times of unfamiliarity and stress. While the idea of keeping piles of work papers and your laptop out of sight seems simple, this habit makes your mind much less likely to wander back to the worries of work. And when it is time to cook and share a meal, you'll feel much more calm and present.

8. Sentimental decorations

Sentimental Decorations - How to Create a Peaceful Home and Peaceful Environment

One way to create a peaceful home is by surrounding yourself with items that are meaningful to you and remind you of a favorite place or time in your life. Our memories are incredible at influencing how we feel. If you love the ocean, choose colors that complement that palette with a fresh accent pillow, a few serene paintings of nature or placing collected seashells in your favorite rooms. Now is the perfect time to refresh with calming interior design and put up a few special family photos.

We are all in this together, and everyone can use a helping hand in creating a peaceful environment in our homes. Small changes to our living spaces can make a big difference. Each of us is adjusting in different ways... we would love to hear how you are creating a more peaceful home!